YOUR KNOWLEDGE HAS VALUE

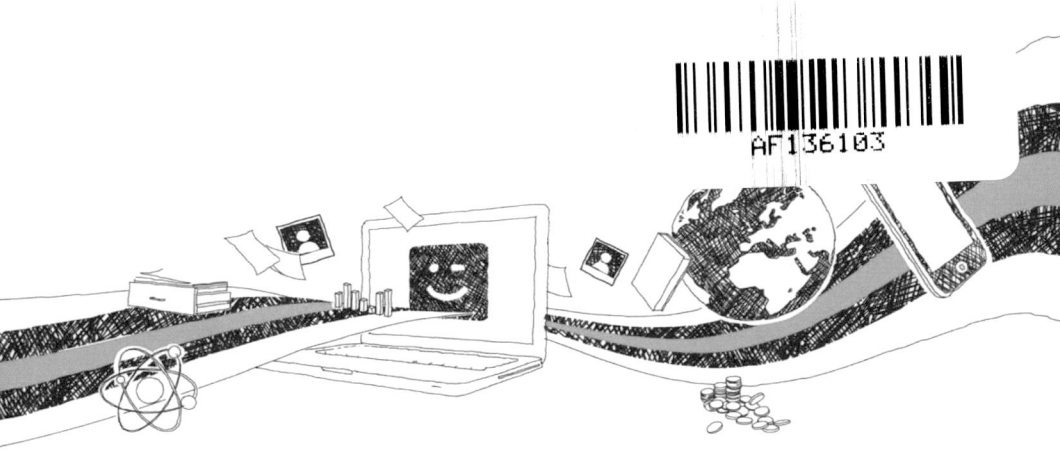

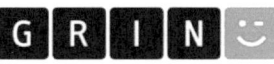

Shirley Murnane

The Occupational Therapy Perspective of Occupation, Health and Well-being

GRIN Publishing

Bibliographic information published by the German National Library:

The German National Library lists this publication in the National Bibliography; detailed bibliographic data are available on the Internet at http://dnb.dnb.de .

Imprint:

Copyright © 2013 GRIN Verlag GmbH
Print and binding: Books on Demand GmbH, Norderstedt Germany
ISBN: 978-3-656-40227-5

This book at GRIN:

http://www.grin.com/en/e-book/211064/the-occupational-therapy-perspective-of-occupation-health-and-well-being

GRIN - Your knowledge has value

Since its foundation in 1998, GRIN has specialized in publishing academic texts by students, college teachers and other academics as e-book and printed book. The website www.grin.com is an ideal platform for presenting term papers, final papers, scientific essays, dissertations and specialist books.

Visit us on the internet:

http://www.grin.com/

http://www.facebook.com/grincom

http://www.twitter.com/grin_com

The Occupational Therapy Perspective of Occupation, Health and Well-being

by

Shirley Murnane

Date of submission: 14/01/2013

The Occupational Therapy Perspective of Occupation, Health and Well-being

This essay begins by briefly introducing some key terms used in occupational therapy (OT) and then discusses how and why the relationship between occupation, health and well-being is so important from the OT perspective. In order to understand this relationship it is necessary to look at the history of the profession and the theory that guides OT practice.

"Occupational therapy enables people to achieve health, well being and life satisfaction through participation in occupation" (College of Occupational Therapy (COT) 2004 as cited in., COT, 2010).

The concept of occupation has evolved throughout the history of the OT profession, as has the centrality of its role (Townsend & Polatajko, 2007). It has proved difficult to reach a clear concise definition of the word occupation, as it must encompass the importance of occupation to human development and experience (Creek, 2010b). In addition, the terms occupation and activity are used interchangeably throughout literature (AOTA, 2008) and some suggest it would be more useful to differentiate between the two terms to improve communication within the profession and with others (Creek, 2010b).

More recently, occupation has been described as the dominant 'activity' of human beings, usually consisting of self-care, work and leisure (Kielhofner, 2009) and as purposeful activity, which engages an individual's time, energy and attention (Reed & Sanderson, 1983). Occupations are composed of skills and values that are meaningful to the person and are influenced by culture and environment (Creek, 2010a). Occupations shape peoples' identity (Christiansen et al., 2005; Duncan, 2006) and are considered necessary for health and wellbeing (Kielhofner, 2009). They engage people in the world and in turn enable survival and self-maintenance (Christiansen et al., 2005). Wilcock (1998) described occupation as an amalgamation of "doing, being and becoming", conceptualising occupation as a dynamic relationship among people's activities of daily life, their occupational nature and their transformation and self-actualisation. These multiple dimensions highlight the complexities that underlie occupation and why it has been difficult to reach a definitive definition (Creek, 2010b).

Activities are the 'doing' process of occupation consisting of a series of goal directed actions that contribute to occupations (Creek, 2010b). Activities do not necessarily hold any meaning for the person (Creek, 2010b), but OT values occupation and activity, as both allow participation in life, and support and maintain health and well-being (AOTA, 2008).

The term health has also lacked a definitive definition. Historically, health has been defined in negative terms focusing only on the absence of disease (Reed and Sanderson, 1999). However, more recently, the World Health Organisation (WHO) (2001) introduced the International Classification of Functioning Disability and Health (ICF), which focuses on how people live with health conditions and can achieve satisfying productive lives (Baum, 2003). It suggests health is an interaction between bodily function, activity engagement and participation as influenced by environmental and personal factors (Baum, 2003). This definition recognises the importance of participation in life, and the negative impact of environmental barriers to occupation on health (Townsend &Polatajko, 2007). This is consistent with the OT perspective, that occupation engagement and participation is fundamental to establishing, maintaining and restoring health (Kielhofner, 2009; Townsend &Polatajko, 2007).

Well-being is a subjective experience that varies between people, consisting of feelings of comfort, pleasure, and health (Schmidt, 2005). Well-being encompasses physical, mental and social dimensions (WHO, 2002 as cited in Wilcock, 1998), extending beyond health to quality of life (Townsend &Polatajko, 2007). People experience well-being when they engage in occupations they perceive as conducive with their values and preferences, which support their plans, goals, occupational identities and their ability to competently perform their valued roles (Townsend &Polatajko, 2007).

Since its inception during the early 20th century the OT profession has been concerned with occupation and its links to health and well-being (Molineux, 2004). The consensus of a profession's core beliefs (Duncan, 2006) is captured in its paradigm, which helps to guide and make sense of practice (Mayers, 2000). The underlying assumptions central to the first OT paradigm were that occupation was a basic human need (Dunton, 1919 as cited in Townsend &Polatajko, 2007), mind and body were linked, and a lack of occupation could result in dysfunction of the mind and body (Keilhofner, 1992). Conversely, occupation had the potential to be therapeutic (Townsend &Polatajko, 2007) restoring health and function (Kielhofner 2009). The person connected to the environment through occupation (Kielhofner, 2009), and occupation was thought of in terms of 'work', which was vital to happiness and wellbeing (Townsend &Polatajko, 2007). Participating in a 'balance of occupations' organised a person's use of time (Meyer, 1992 cited in Letts et al., 2003) and brought structure to living (Townsend &Polatajko, 2007). The paradigm valued holism and recognised the importance of occupation and its links to health and human dignity (Duncan, 2006). People were viewed as occupational beings, with the right to engage in meaningful occupation (Kielhofner, 2009) and the focus of the profession was on intrinsic motivation and the effect of the environment on occupational performance (Duncan, 2006).

Towards the middle of the 20th century OT was transferred to the 'Medical Division" civil service classification from the 'Trades and Industries' (Gritzer&Arluke, 1985 as cited in Hopkins & Smith, 1993) thus, aligning OT more closely to the medical profession (Hopkins & Smith, 1993). This alliance placed increasing pressure on OT to be more objective, and to create a theoretical rationale for its intervention, inline with medicine's scientific view (Kielhofner, 2009). During this period the OT profession gained a deeper understanding of how body structures and functions influence performance, and technological advances in the use of aids and adaptive devices for remediating impairments and adapting the environment (Kielhofner, 2009). The OT profession began to focus on biomedical explanations for practice in an attempt to gain professional acceptance and thus the mechanistic paradigm was born (Duncan, 2006). The assumptions of the profession were that occupational performance was dependent on the integrity of internal body systems, damage or abnormal development of any one of these systems could cause dysfunction, and functional limitations could be restored using compensatory methods (Molineux, 2004). The person and the environment were viewed as separate elements (Letts, et al., 2003) and risk factors in the environment were thought to contribute to the process of disease, but the disease itself was said to rest within the person (Reed and Sanderson, 1999). Occupation was used to address and measure impaired inner systems (Duncan, 2006). People were seen as passive recipients of treatment and therapy was applied to the impaired body parts, rather than viewing the person as an integrated whole who can act upon the environment (Hopkins and Smith, 1993) and an occupational perspective was largely lost (Molineux, 2004).

The embracement of the reductionist approach was recognised as insufficient by prominent figures within the OT profession such as Occupational Therapist Mary Reilly, who in 1962, called for the profession to return to its roots and to recommit to a focus on occupation (Reilly, 1962 as cited in., Kielhofner, 2009). Reilly (1962) as cited in Kielhofner (2009), stated that " man, through the use of his hands as they are energised by mind and will can influence the state of his own health". This

4

reaffirmation reflected the most seminal ideas of the profession that people are active agents who can improve, maintain or restore their occupational performance and health (Hopkins & Smith, 1993). Reilly was concerned that the fragmented knowledge used by the profession from diverse disciplines, could displace the understanding of occupation, and she felt that the profession needed consistency and unity of theoretical knowledge (Hopkins and Smith, 1993). The uniqueness of the OT perspective was becoming blurred due to its adaptability within healthcare to fit the needs of the day (Wilcock, 2001) and being unique is a hallmark of a true profession (Reilly, 1958 as cited in., Molineux, 2004). During this period there was a resurgence of interest in occupation, and recognition of the important interaction between the person, environment and occupation on occupational performance, health and well-being (Letts et al., 2003), and the contemporary paradigm began to emerge.

The core assumptions of the emerging contemporary paradigm are that people are occupational by nature, barriers to occupation impact on health and wellbeing, and occupation can be used as a therapeutic tool (Kielhofner, 2009). The paradigm recognises the value of human life, engagement in occupation, peoples right to have choice control and in their occupations, and social integration through meaningful occupation (Duncan, 2006). Knowledge gained from both the aforementioned paradigms is incorporated in the contemporary paradigm; the influence of performance components on occupation, technological knowledge of adaptive devices, the centrality of occupation and the recognition that the person is connected to the environment (Kielhofner, 2009). Occupation and holism are the focus of the paradigm (Duncan, 2006).

Occupational therapists working in the modern health and social care service can find addressing the occupational needs of people problematic, often due to factors such as the dominance of the medical model, coupled with political, institutional and financial pressures (Molineux, 2004). Some suggest that the survival of the profession has been due to it's 'usefulness' (Creek, 1999 as cited in., Fortune, 2000) and adoption of a reductionist approach, but as a result therapists have become philosophically lost, failing to use the OT framework to guide practice and assert a unique OT identity (Fortune, 2000).

The OT practice framework (AOTA, 2008) is based on the philosophy of the contemporary paradigm and outlines the profession's scope of practice and areas of expert knowledge, which form the OT domain of concern. Therapists use the framework to guide them during practice (AOTA, 2008). The framework identifies six aspects of the OT domain: Areas of occupation; client factors; performance skills; performance patterns; context and environment; features and demands of activity, which influence engagement, participation and health (AOTA, 2008).

The main focus of the domain is the areas of occupation which consist of: activities of daily living; instrumental activities of daily living; education; work; play; leisure; and social participation (AOTA, 2008). Occupational therapists use the framework to support people to achieve occupational justice, people can experience occupational injustice due to personal and societal factors, which act as barriers to occupation, leading to occupational imbalance, deprivation or alienation (Townsend &Wilcock, 2004 as cited in Townsend &Polatajko, 2007). Occupational imbalance is a lack of balance between work, rest, and play, which can result in poorer health, decreased life satisfaction and well-being (Townsend &Polatajko, 2007). The term occupational deprivation is used to describe an enduring restriction in the ability to participate in meaningful occupations, due to barriers in the multi dimensional environment, which can undermine health and well-being (Townsend &Polatajko, 2007). Occupational alienation refers to feelings of powerlessness in the ability to change one's situation, and a lack of meaning or sense of fulfilment in one's occupations (Hagedorn, 2001 as cited in Creek, 2010).

Occupational identity has a powerful motivational influence on participation in occupation, and is generated from the person's occupational performance history, a sense of who the person is, and aspires to become (Duncan, 2006). Occupational identity consists of: a sense of the person, as defined by their roles and relationships; their performance patterns; sense of self efficacy; their interests, obligations and beliefs, (Duncan 2006) and their spirituality (connection with self, others, nature and a higher power or source of ultimate meaning) (Christiansen et al., 2005).

Performance skills refer to the components of performance; the observable abilities in the actions people perform (AOTA, 2008). Performance skills have been categorised as: motor and praxis; sensory-perceptual; emotion regulation; cognitive and communication and social skills (AOTA, 2008). Underlying body functions and structures reflect the person's internal capacity and performance skills reflect the person's demonstrated abilities, which influence performance. Performance skills are closely related and can be used in conjunction with one another and a change in the performance of one skill can affect another (AOTA, 2008). Context, activity demands and the person's body functions and structures, may serve to support or hinder acquisition or demonstration of performance skills (AOTA, 2008).

Daily occupations are organised into habitual patterns of behaviour, which are governed by our habits, roles (Duncan, 2006) and routines, which structure daily life (AOTA, 2008). Performance patterns are influenced by all aspects of the domain, and develop over time (AOTA, 2008). Habits refer to the automatic thoughts and actions (Christiansen et al., 2005), which regulate our behaviour on a daily basis (Duncan, 2006). Habits can be useful for example helping to reduce mental and physical effort when responding to unfolding situations, allowing attention to be divided effectively (Dewey, 1922 as cited in Christiansen et al., 2005). Conversely, habits can be impoverished, as found in people with depression and attention disorders, or dominating as found in addictive behaviours (Dunn, 2000 as cited in Christiansen et al., 2005).

Routines refer to the established repetitive patterns of occupations or activities, which provide structure (AOTA, 2008) and maintain daily life (Clark, 2000 as cited in Christiansen et al., 2005). Disruption to routine can lead to occupational deprivation as found when sleep patterns are interrupted; sleep is a necessary routine for self-maintenance and survival (Aronoff, 1991 as cited in Christiansen et al., 2005). Roles influence the occupations and associated activities people engage in (Keilhofner, 1995), they are dynamic changing throughout the lifespan (Christiansen et al., 2005) and have social norms, which are shaped by culture and defined by the person (AOTA, 2008). Changes in roles and environment can lead to occupational disruption and occupational alienation, resulting in psychological and physical consequences, as found when individuals are institutionalised or homeless (Whiteford, 1995 as cited in Christiansen et al., 2005).

Therapists use their expert knowledge to evaluate performance issues in any or all of the areas of the domain during the OT process (AOTA, 2008), to guide people through environmental and personal change during life transitions, and to develop healthy habits of occupation (CAOT, 2008). The OT process consists of a series of circuitous actions, with stages that combine and overlap (Duncan, 2006). Creek (2003) describes 11 stages: referral or reason for contact; information gathering; initial interview; reason for intervention/needs identification/problem formulation; set goals; action plan; action; ongoing assessment; outcome and outcome measurement; end of intervention or discharge followed by a final review (Creek, 2003).

Conceptual models of OT help to organise the theoretical assumptions of the profession and domain of concern (Turpin &Iwama, 2009) and provide explanations of the dynamic relationship between the person, occupation, and the environment, which guide practice during the OT process (Duncan, 2006).   A model used throughout the profession is the Canadian Model of Occupational Performance and Engagement (CMOP-E) (Polatajko et al., 2007), which is a revision of the Canadian Model of Occupational Performance (CMOP) (CAOT 1997 as cited in., Townsend &Polatajko, 2007). The CMOP-E is a client-centred model, which recognises the importance of individual empowerment and engagement to occupation, and views the person as connected to the environment through occupation (Townsend &Polatajko, 2007). The model specifies 3 elements: Occupation, consisting of self-care, leisure and productivity; the person consisting of physical, affective and cognitive performance and engagement components, with spirituality at the core and the multidimensional environment consisting of cultural, institutional, physical and social dimensions (Townsend &Polatajko, 2007). Occupation is the means by which the person interacts with, and acts upon their environment; disruption to any one element can affect all others, resulting in occupational injustice (Townsend &Polatajko, 2007).

The CMOP-E states it is important to establish a client-therapist relationship to form a trusting environment, and to develop an understanding of each other's occupational nature (Townsend &Polatajko, 2007). At the point of referral, the therapist makes contact with the client to identify reasons for referral, and to ascertain the clients' readiness to change (Townsend &Polatajko, 2007). The clients' occupational status, environmental and personal factors are evaluated during the initial assessment and the findings are interpreted to establish explanations for occupational issues and formulate recommendations (Townsend &Polatajko, 2007). The Canadian Occupational Performance Measure (COPM) (Law et al., 2005 as cited in., Townsend &Polatajko, 2007) is an assessment tool developed for use with the model, which can be used to gain a baseline measure following the initial assessment to establish the clients' self-perception of occupational performance and level of satisfaction using a self-rating scale. The client also rates the importance of each occupation, which can be used to identify and prioritise goals for intervention with the therapist (Townsend &Polatajko, 2007). The therapist helps the client to choose achievable and realistic goals and they collaborate to formulate a plan for intervention (Townsend &Polatajko, 2007). The clients' progress can be re-evaluated throughout the intervention using the COPM, to measure change in the clients' perceived level of performance and satisfaction, and modifications can be made if issues arise or progress is slow (Townsend &Polatajko, 2007). Once the client has no ongoing occupational issues and identified goals have been met the COPM is re-administered to obtain an outcome measure, and the intervention is evaluated (Townsend &Polatajko, 2007). If goals have not been met or the client has other occupational issues, new objectives can be set or the process can be concluded and the client discharged (Townsend &Polatajko, 2007).

In conclusion, it is apparent that the OT perspective of occupation, health and well-being has evolved throughout the history of the profession, as reflected in its paradigms. OT recognises the importance of the relationship between occupation, health and well-being and is focused on supporting participation of meaningful occupation, individual empowerment and in promoting occupational justice. OT has continued to widen its knowledge and scope, and therapists currently work in various areas of health and social care. However, for the profession to continue to develop it must seek new opportunities to provide a service to those who face barriers to occupation in modern society (Parnell & Wilding, 2010). In addition, it is imperative that therapists keep up to date with OT theory to guide practice, and remember where they have come from to assert a unique OT identity (Fortune, 2000).

Reference List

American Occupational Therapy Association. (2008) Occupational therapy practice framework: Domain and process. *American Journal of Occupational Therapy*. 62 (6), 625-683.

Baum, M. C. (2003) Participation: it's relationship to occupation and health. *OTJR: Occupation, Participation and Health*, 23(2), 46-47.

Canadian Association of Occupational Therapists. (2008) *CAOT Position Statement: Occupations and Health*. Retrieved January 5, 2013 from http://www.caot.ca/pdfs/positionstate/occhealth.pdf

Christiansen, C. H., Baum, C. M. and J. Bass-Haugen (Eds.) (2005) *Occupational Therapy Performance, Participation, and Well-Being* (3rd Ed.). Thorofare, NJ: Slack

College of Occupational Therapists (2010) *Code of Ethics and Professional Conduct*. London: COT.

Creek, J. (2003) *Occupational therapy defined as a complex intervention*. London: College of Occupational Therapists

Creek, J. (2010a) Culturally and socially significant activity. *South African Journal of Occupational Therapy –Supplement*, August, pp2-4

Creek, J. (2010b) *The Core Concepts of Occupational Therapy: A Dynamic Framework for Practice*. Jessica Kingsley

Duncan, E. AS. (Ed) (2006) *Foundations for Practice in Occupational Therapy* (4th Ed). London: Elsevier

Fortune, T. (2000) Occupational therapists: is our Therapy truly Occupational or are we merely filling gaps? *British Journal of Occupational Therapy*, 63(5), 225-230.

Hagedorn, R. (2001) *Occupational Therapy: Perspectives and Processes*. London: Churchill Livingstone.

Hopkins, H. L., & Smith, H. D. (1993) *Willard and Spackman's Occupational Therapy* (8th Ed). USA: J. B. Lippincott Company.

Kielhofner, G. (2009) *Conceptual Foundations of Occupational Therapy* (4th Ed). FA Davis: Philadelphia.

Law, M., Stanton, S., Polatajko, H., Baptiste, S., Thompson- Franson, T., Kramer, C., Swedlove, F., Brintnell, S., & Campanile, L. (1997) *Enabling Occupation: an occupational therapy perspective.* Ottawa: CAOT Publications

Letts, L., Rigby, P., & Stewart, D. (2003) *Using Environments to Enable Occupational Performance.* Thorofare, NJ: Slack.

Mayers, C. A. (2000) The Casson Memorial Lecture 2000: Reflect on the past to Shape the Future. *British Journal of Occupational Therapy,* 63(8), 358-366.

Molineux, M. (2004) *Occupation in occupational therapy: A labour in vain?* In M. Molineux (Ed.), *Occupation for Occupational Therapists* (pp 1-14). Oxford: Blackwell Publishing.

Parnell, T., Wilding, C. (2010) Where can occupation-focussed philosophy take occupational therapy? *Australian Occupational Therapy Journal,* 57(5), 345-348.

Polatajko, H.J., Townsend, E.A. &Craik, J. (2007) Canadian Model of Occupational Performance and Engagement (CMOP-E). In *Enabling occupation II: Advancing an occupational therapy vision for health, well-being, & justice through occupation.* Ottawa, ON: CAOT Publications ACE. 22-36.

Reed. K. L., & Sanderson, S. N. (1999) *Concepts of occupational therapy* (4th Ed). Philadelphia, PA: Lippincott Williams and Wilkins.

Schmid, T. (2005) Promoting health through creativity: an introduction. In: Schmid, T. (ed) *Promoting health through creativity for professionals in health, arts and education,* Whurr, London.

Townsend, E.A., &Polatajko, H.J. (2007) *Enabling occupation II: Advancing an occupational therapy vision for health, well-being, & justice through occupation.* Ottawa, ON: CAOT.

Turpin, M. J., &Iwama, M. K. (2009) Using Occupational Therapy Models in Practice (1st Ed): A Field guide. Edinburgh: Churchill Livingstone Elsevier.

Wilcock, A. (1998) Reflections on doing, being and becoming.*Canadian Journal of Occupational Therapy,* 65, 248–256.

Wilcock, A. (2001) Occupational Science: the Key to Broadening Horizons. *British Journal of Occupational Therapy,* 64(8), 412-417.

Wilcock, A. (2006) *An Occupational Perspective of Health* (2nd Ed) Thorofare, NJ: Slack.